Strong at Sixty:

Core Exercises to Keep Seniors Fit and Healthy.

BY

Jennifer Danielson

TABLE OF CONTENT

Introduction

Hello, and thank you for joining us here at "Strong at Sixty: Core Exercises to Keep Seniors Fit and Healthy." The exercises in this book are designed to help elderly citizens over 60 build their core strength safely and effectively. The human body goes through several changes as we age, including the gradual loss of bone density and muscle mass. Exercises that focus on the abdominal muscles are an integral part of a healthy lifestyle and can assist senior citizens in preserving their independence and quality of life.

In this book, you will learn why it is so important for seniors to have core strength, how to evaluate your current core strength, and how to design a specialized workout program tailored to your unique requirements and fitness level. We will also go through the most effective core exercises for older adults and adjustments and progressions for people of varying fitness levels. We will also discuss how to keep your core strength over your lifetime.

This book is meant to equip you with the tools and information to stay strong and healthy as you age, regardless of whether you are an experienced athlete or just starting with exercise. Now that we have everything out let's begin your journey to a better and healthier you!

Why Older People need to Do Core Exercises

Exercises that focus on the core are essential for people of advanced age since they help to preserve strength, balance, and stability. The muscles and bones in our bodies naturally weaken as we age, making us more susceptible to injuries such as fractures, broken bones, and other accidents. Your ability to strengthen the muscles that support your spine and pelvis, improve your posture, and boost your available balance and stability can all be accomplished by including core exercises as part of your regular workout program.

Your capacity to carry out activities of daily living, such as getting out of a chair or reaching for an item on a high shelf, will increase as a direct result of your participation in core exercises. When you have strong core muscles, you are less likely to feel pain or discomfort in your back, hips, or other areas. This is because your core muscles support your spine and provide stability.

In addition, activities that focus on your core benefit your mental and emotional well-being. It is well-known that physical activity can improve mood and lower stress levels; feeling physically strong and capable can enhance your general sense of well-being.

Including core workouts in your routine can substantially impact your health and quality of life as you age. This is especially true if you start doing those activities later in life.

Tips and Tricks to Help You Get the Most Out of This Book

It is essential to enter this book with an open mind and the desire to attempt new activities and strategies to maximize its offers. The following are some suggestions that will assist you in getting the most out of your time spent reading:

1. Read the book all the way through to understand better the significance of core strength and how it connects to your overall health as a senior. This will help you better grasp the value of core strength and how it relates to your overall health.

2. Take notes: As you read the book, write down any critical points that jump out at you. This will assist you in remembering the material and exercises most essential to you.

3. Putting these exercises into practice is the most effective way to enhance your core strength, and they are

detailed in detail throughout this book. Spend the time necessary to complete each exercise, paying close attention to your form and technique as you go.

4. It is crucial to start slowly and gradually increase the difficulty of your workouts over time. If you are new to fitness or last worked on your core a while ago, it is necessary to start slowly and progressively growing the depth of your workouts. Please pay attention to what your body tells you, and stop what you're doing when necessary.

5. Don't be afraid to ask for assistance: If you are unsure about a specific activity or have questions about your fitness level, feel free to ask for help. A trained fitness professional may direct you through the movements of the exercises and assist you in developing a personalized training program tailored to your specific requirements. You may get the most out of "Strong at Sixty: Core Exercises to Keep Seniors Fit and Healthy" and enhance your general health and well-being as you age by

following these guidelines and getting the most out of the book .

Chapter 1

Understanding Core Strength

We will discuss what core strength is, why it is essential for seniors, and how it influences tasks that people do daily. What exactly does "core strength" mean? The muscles that make up the boot of your body, including those in your belly, back, and pelvis, are referred to collectively as your core.

Core strength is an essential factor in overall fitness. These muscles collaborate to support your spine, aid in maintaining proper posture, and make it easier for you to move your body.

Why Maintaining a Strong Core Is Important for Seniors

Keeping excellent core strength is especially crucial for seniors, as it can help prevent injuries and falls that can occur more frequently. The muscles and bones in our bodies naturally weaken as we age, making us more susceptible to injuries such as broken bones and fall. By helping to improve balance and stability, which minimizes the chance of losing, having strong core muscles can be beneficial. In addition, having a solid core can aid in increasing your capacity to carry out day-to-day activities such as getting out of a chair, lifting groceries, or reaching for an item that is stored on a high shelf. When you have strong core muscles, you are less likely to feel pain or discomfort in your back, hips, or other areas. This is because your core muscles support your spine and provide stability.

How Core Strength Affects Things You Do Daily.
The strength of your abdominal muscles is an essential factor in many of the tasks you carry out daily. For instance, when you leave a chair, your abdominal muscles stabilize your body and support your spine so you don't fall over. When you walk, the core muscles in your body are put to work to keep your posture and balance in check. Even routine tasks, such as bending over to tie your shoes

or reaching for an item on a higher shelf, require adequate core strength. You can begin to appreciate the value of including core exercises in your fitness regimen after you have a grasp of the significance of core strength and how it influences activities that are performed daily.

In the following chapter, we will discuss how to evaluate your core strength and identify the types of workouts that will be most beneficial for you.

What exactly does "core strength" mean?

Core strength is the ability of the muscles in your belly, back, and pelvis to function in unison to stabilize your spine, keep your posture in check, and make it easier for you to move your body. These muscles maintain your body's stability while driving and engaging in tasks like walking, bending, twisting, and lifting.Building middle electricity can assist enhance your balance, stability, and coordination, that could assist decrease the hazard of damage from falls. In addition, having a solid core can help reduce or prevent pain and discomfort in other body parts, including the back, the hips, and different body sections. Core strength benefits people of all ages but becomes more significant as we age. Seniors can improve their overall quality of life by keeping adequate core strength, which allows them to improve their balance and stability, minimizing the danger of falling and enhancing their overall quality of life. Core strength is essential to a healthy and active lifestyle, and incorporating core exercises into your regular workout routine can significantly benefit your physical and mental well-being. In general, core strength is essential to a healthy and active lifestyle.

How Core Strength Affects Things You Do Daily

Core strength influences day-to-day activity in a variety of different ways. The following are some examples:

1.Getting up from a chair The use of core muscles helps to support the body when getting up from a chair, which not only makes the movement simpler but also lowers the chance of falling.

2.When you walk, the muscles in your core are engaged to help you keep a healthy posture and maintain your balance. This can help lower the chance of tripping or falling.

3.Object lifting engages the core muscles, stabilizing the spine and limiting the likelihood of injury. This is especially important when lifting heavy objects.

4.When reaching for things, having strong core muscles helps support the body, making the activity more straightforward and lowering the chance of falling over or losing your equilibrium.

5.As you bend over to pick something up, you engage the core muscles in your body, which helps to stabilize the body and prevents strain on the lower back.

Strong core muscles make it easier to conduct daily life tasks, lowering the chance of injury and improving overall physical function. Seniors can preserve their independence and continue carrying out the abovementioned studies with relative ease if they strengthen their core strengths.

Cautionary Measures and Advice for Seniors About Core Exercises

Some precautions and safety measures should be kept in mind to limit the chance of harm when engaging in core exercises; nonetheless, core workouts are generally safe and helpful for seniors.

1.Talk to Your Doctor Before Beginning an Exercise Program It is always a good idea to talk to your doctor before beginning any fitness program. This is especially important if you have any pre-existing health concerns.

2.If you are new to fitness or last worked out a while ago, begin with less complicated exercises and work up to more difficult ones as you progress. Start slow and work your way up.

3. Use the Correct Form: Correct form is vital to avoiding injury and efficiently engaging the core muscles in any exercise. Be sure to follow the instructions carefully, and if you have any questions, feel free to ask for clarification.

4.Prevent Overexertion: Don't put too much pressure on yourself; avoid workouts that hurt or make you uncomfortable. Please pay attention to what your body tells you and give it the necessary breaks.

5.Make Sure Your Equipment Is Appropriate If you're using equipment like an exercise ball or a resistance band, be sure it's the right size for you and has the right amount of resistance for your goals.

6.Maintain Your Hydration Levels: Before, during, and after your workout, make sure you drink lots of water to avoid becoming dehydrated.

7.Think About Working with a Trainer If you need help performing particular exercises or desire more individualized coaching, think about working with a qualified personal trainer or physical therapist.

Chapter 2

Evaluating Your Core Strength

In the second chapter, we will go through how to evaluate your abdominal strength. This is a crucial first step in establishing a core fitness program personalized to your requirements and capabilities.

In this session, we will discuss the following topics:

1.Why it is essential to evaluate your abdominal and back strength

2.Core strength can be evaluated using a variety of approaches, including self-evaluation and collaboration with a trained professional.

3.Learn to locate problematic areas of your core muscles, whether they are areas of weakness or instability

4.How to keep track of your improvements over time and adapt your workout routine accordingly

At the end of this chapter, you will have a better awareness of your current level of core strength and be able to design a more effective exercise program personalized to your particular needs and goals. You will also have the ability to develop a more effective exercise program..

How to Determine Whether Your Core Strength Is Adequate

There are a few different ways to measure an individual's core strength. Here are several examples:

1.Self-evaluation: To get started, all you have to do is pay attention to how the muscles in your core feel while you go about your daily activities. When you walk or get up from a chair, do you have a sense that you are stable and balanced? Do you suffer from pain or discomfort in the region of your lower back? These are possible indications of fundamental flaws.

2.The plank test is a popular exercise to evaluate abdominal and back strength. To begin, get into the plank position by placing your forearms on the ground and lining up your body so that it is in a straight line. It would help if you maintained this position for as long as possible. Your core muscles will be more vital if you keep the plank position longer.

3.The leg lowering test requires you to lie on your back with your legs raised straight. While maintaining a standing position with both legs, move one leg down toward the ground in a controlled manner. Your core strength is vital if you can perform the exercise in which you lower one knee toward the floor without arching your back. If you notice that your back is starting to arch, you may have weak core muscles.

4.Working with a fitness professional or a physical therapist can provide a more comprehensive test of your core strength than assessing it alone. They might use electromyography (EMG) to evaluate muscle activation during exercises or a functional movement screen (FMS) to analyze general movement patterns.

If you first evaluate your core strength, you can build a more targeted workout program to increase your general strength and function. This will allow you to identify areas of weakness or imbalance in your body.

Concerns that the Elderly Have in Common About Their Core Strength

Problems regarding our core strength may arise as we get older. The following are some common difficulties related to core strength that seniors may encounter:

1.The age-related decrease of muscular mass known as sarcopenia, commonly known as sarcopenia, can cause the abdominal muscles to become weaker.

2.Bad posture can be caused by years of sitting, standing, and moving poorly, leading to weak and imbalanced core muscles.

3.Injuries that occurred in the past: Injuries that occurred in the past, such as surgery, can lead to muscular imbalances and weakening in the core.

4.A sedentary lifestyle with no physical activity can weaken core muscles and general physical weakness.

5.Stable conditions: Long-lasting Conditions, such as arthritis or osteoporosis, can impact core strength and total physical function.

To build an effective workout program that targets the underlying difficulties contributing to issues with core strength, it is vital to identify any underlying concerns contributing to those issues. Increase both your core strength and your total physical function by concentrating on workouts for core strength that are tailored to the specific requirements and capabilities of the individual.

When to Seek the Assistance of a Professional

Suppose you experience any pain or discomfort while exercising or participating in everyday activities and any underlying medical disorders that may influence your ability to exercise safely. In that case, you must seek the assistance of a trained professional.

In addition, if you are new to exercise or have not exercised regularly for a long time, it may be helpful to work with a fitness professional or physical therapist to ensure that you are using the correct form and technique, as well as to develop a safe and effective exercise program that is tailored to your individual needs and abilities. If you are new to exercise or have not exercised regularly for a long time, working with a fitness professional or physical therapist may be helpful.

When beginning a new fitness program, it is always a good idea to speak with your healthcare practitioner if you have concerns about your core strength or physical function. This is especially important if you have been inactive for an extended period. They will be able to direct you in the right direction and make suggestions depending on your medical history and current physical health state.

Chapter 3

Beginning Your Core Workout Routine

This chapter will discuss the fundamentals of starting an exercise program focusing on the core. These are the following:

1.Creating attainable objectives: In this section, we will explore how to develop goals within your reach, which will help you remain motivated and measure your progress.

2.Selecting the Right Exercises: In this section, we will present an overview of some of the most effective core exercises for seniors, including variations for different fitness levels and physical abilities.

3.Developing a strategy for your workouts: We will provide direction on how to structure your workouts, including how often you should exercise and strike a balance between core exercises and other forms of physical activity.

4.Important safety factors, such as correct form and technique, as well as information on how to avoid harm, will be discussed in this section.

By the conclusion of this chapter, you will be equipped with the knowledge and resources necessary to initiate a safe, efficient core fitness program that suits your specific requirements and objectives.

The Process of Getting Your Body Ready for Workout

Getting your body ready for any fitness program before beginning is essential, as this will help you avoid injury and get the most out of your sessions at the gym. The following is a list of suggestions for getting your body ready for exercise:

1.It would help to begin with a warm-up to prepare your muscles and joints for activity. You must perform a proper introduction. To get your heart rate up and your blood flowing, you should begin with five to ten minutes of modest cardiovascular exercise, such as walking or cycling.

2.After you've finished your warm-up, stretching your muscles for a few minutes is essential. Concentrate on the primary muscle groups, such as your hamstrings, quadriceps, and core muscles, that you will be working on during your workout, such as running or lifting weights. Each stretch should be held for fifteen to thirty seconds, and you should avoid bouncing or straining the space.

3. Keep yourself hydrated by drinking lots of water before, during, and after your workout to avoid dehydration and ensure you get the most out of your activity.

4.Put on clothing and footwear that are suitable for the activity you have selected. This includes comfortable, breathable clothing and shoes that provide adequate support.

5.Please pay attention to how your body feels while you work out, and be sure to give it the attention it deserves. You should immediately stop what you're doing and rest if you feel pain, discomfort, or shortness of breath. It is critical to begin your workouts at a low intensity and progressively build up both the duration and difficulty level as you progress.

You can maximize the benefits of your exercises and lower the likelihood of suffering an injury if you take the time to do the things necessary to get your body ready for training.

Establishing Objectives That Can Be Met

While beginning a program of core exercises, it is crucial to create goals that are practical and relevant to you and that you can achieve. Here are some tips for setting goals:

1.Determine what you want to accomplish: do you wish to enhance your posture, lessen the pain in your back, or boost your overall strength and fitness level? Having clear objectives in mind will make it easier for you to maintain your motivation and focus on what you wish to accomplish.

2.Make sure that your goals are clear and concise. Too general objectives, such as "getting in shape" or "reducing weight," might be challenging. Ensure your goals are well-defined and measurable, such as "increasing my core strength by 20 percent in the next three months."

3.Make sure to let the prospect of achieving your goals overwhelm you; instead, take the time to break them into more manageable chunks. You may work on them daily or weekly if you break them down into smaller, more manageable steps first.

4.Be practical: When you set objectives for yourself, ensure they are challenging but still doable, given your current fitness level and lifestyle. If you create goals that are too difficult to achieve, you risk being disheartened and giving up.

5.Maintain tabs on your progression: One of the best ways to keep tabs on your progression is to document your workouts and analyze how well you are doing. This can make it easier for you to maintain your motivation and appreciate your accomplishments.

You'll be able to keep yourself motivated and focused on improving your core strength and fitness if you set attainable and relevant goals.

Developing a Strategy for Your Exercise Routine

A plan for your core exercises is a vital step in starting a fitness routine. The following are some suggestions for developing an efficient method for your workouts:

1. Try to perform core exercises between two and three times per week, allowing at least one day of rest between each set of activities.

2. **Duration:**

   1. Begin with shorter workouts and progressively increase the course as you grow more familiar with the exercises.

   2. Start with shorter workouts and work your way up to longer workouts.

   3. Aim for doing core exercises for 10 to 15 minutes per session, and work your way up to doing them for 30 minutes or longer.

3. Exercises: Choose a range of activities that work the primary muscle groups in your core, such as your abdominals, lower back, and obliques. Use a variety of

core exercises in your workout routine, such as planks, crunches, and bridges, to ensure that you are effectively targeting all of the core muscle groups.

4.Sets and Reps: To begin, perform one to two sets of each exercise, with eight to twelve repetitions in each group. As your strength improves, the number of sets and reps you perform should also gradually rise.

5.Rest: Give yourself a few minutes to relax and recover between each set. Aim for a rest period of thirty to sixty seconds between each group.

6.The progression calls for you to gradually ramp up the intensity and difficulty of your workouts as you continue to get stronger. Increasing the length of your exercises, the number of sets and reps you perform, and the amount of weight or resistance you use are all examples.

Always remember to remember what your body tells you and adapt your exercise routine accordingly. If you are experiencing any pain or discomfort, you should immediately stop what you are doing and talk to a medical expert.

Chapter 4

The Most Effective Core Exercises for Older Adults

Starting Exercises to Get You Warmed Up and Stretched Out

It is crucial to warm up your muscles and get your body ready for physical activity before going into core workouts. The following are some activities for warming up and stretching that may be helpful:

1.Exercises for the neck include tilting your head to one side while holding the position for ten to fifteen seconds and then repeating the stretch on the other side. After that, tilt your head forward and hold this position for ten to fifteen seconds. After that, tilt your head back and hold this position for the same length.

2.Shoulder Rotations Start by rotating your shoulders forward in a circular motion, then roll them backward. Continue in this manner for 10–15 repetitions.

3.Exercise your arms by moving them in short circles in front of and behind your body by extending them to the sides. Start with little circles and work up to larger ones until you can complete entire revolutions.

4.Torso Twists: While standing with your feet shoulder-width apart, twist your torso to one side, then back to the center, and then to the other side. Repeat this movement three times. Continue in this manner for 10–15 repetitions.

5.To perform hip circles, stand with your feet about shoulder-width apart and move your hips clockwise and anticlockwise while making circles with them.

6.Stand with your feet about shoulder-width apart to perform knee lifts and bring one knee up towards your chest. After getting it back down to the starting position, epeat the movement on the other side. Continue in this manner for 10–15 repetitions.

Remember to begin your workout with easy motions and gradually build the intensity as your muscles warm up. Seniors can enhance their core strength through various exercises, which can be found online. The following are some of the most effective core workouts for older adults:

1.Exercises using the plank position are excellent for developing the entire core, including the abdominal muscles, the lower back, and the oblique muscles. Start in a push-up place and hold your body in a straight line while keeping your elbows and forearms on the ground. This is the beginning position for the plank.

2.Crunches: Crunches are a time-honored core workout that can assist seniors in developing stronger abdominal muscles. Lie on your back with your legs bent and your hands behind your head. This position will allow you to perform a crunch. Raise your shoulders and tense your core to complete the exercise.

3.Bridges are an excellent workout for strengthening the lower back and the glutes. Lie on your back with your knees bent and your feet planted firmly on the ground. This is the starting position for a bridge. Raise your hips off the ground while contracting your glutes during the movement.

4.Obliques can be significantly strengthened with the help of Russian twists, which are excellent exercises. To execute a Russian twist, you should begin by sitting on the ground with your knees bent and your feet planted firmly on the floor. Lean back just a little bit and twist your torso to the side, being sure to touch the ground with one hand. On the other side, repeat the process.

5. Planches latérales: Les planches latérales sont un excellent exercice pour renforcer les abdominaux et améliorer la balance. Beginning in the plank position,

swivel your body to one side while supporting yourself on one elbow and the side of one foot. This is a side plank.

6.Bird dog: The bird dog exercise is fantastic for building strength in the lower back and improving balance. Beginning on your hands and knees, perform a bird dog by extending one arm and the leg that is diagonally opposite it. Hold this position for a few seconds before switching sides.

As a senior, you can increase your core strength and general fitness by including the activities in your regular core workout routine. Remember that you should begin your workouts leisurely and progressively raise the intensity and difficulty of your exercises as your strength increases.

An Overview of the Many-Core Workout Varieties Available

An Introduction to the Many Varieties of Core Exercises:

1.Isometric exercises are exercises in which the participant maintains a static position for a predetermined time. Some examples of this would be planks as well as side planks.

2.Exercises that incorporate movement and help increase mobility and flexibility are called dynamic exercises. Dynamic exercises help enhance mobility and flexibility. Crunches and Russian twists are two examples of exercises.

3.Stability exercises help enhance one's balance and coordination. Stability exercises help improve balance. The bird dog and the single-leg balance are just two examples.

4.Resistance exercises entail adding weight or resistance to an existing routine to increase the difficulty of the exercise and improve strength. Examples of this type of exercise include cable rotations and weighted crunches.

5.Yoga and Pilates: Both yoga and Pilates are forms of low-impact exercise that can assist in increasing one's core strength and flexibility. Planks in yoga and Pilates, as well as spinal twists, are some examples of core-strengthening exercises.

6.Aerobic exercises: Aerobic exercises, such as jogging, cycling, and swimming, can help build core strength. Core muscles support the body during movement. Thus strengthening those muscles can assist in enhancing overall stability.

You may improve your general fitness and mobility as a senior by incorporating a number of these different sorts of core exercises into your training program. This can help you build a solid and balanced core and improve your overall fitness.

The Best Abdominal Workouts for Seniors

1.Exercises using the plank position are excellent for developing the entire core, including the abdominal muscles, the lower back, and the oblique muscles. For those who are just starting, it is recommended that you perform them on your forearms or hands and knees.

2.Bridges are an excellent workout for strengthening the lower back and the glutes. Alternatively, you can increase the difficulty level by adding resistance by inserting a ball or cushion in the space between your knees.

3.The "Bird Dog" exercise is fantastic for building strength in the lower back and increasing balance, and it's named appropriately. Beginning on your hands and knees, perform a bird dog by extending one arm and the leg that is diagonally opposite it. Hold this position for a few seconds before switching sides.

4.Exercises such as the wall sit are fantastic for building strength in the lower body and the abdominal region. Stand with your back against a wall and slide down until your knees are bent at a 90-degree angle to do a wall sit.

5.Standing Balance: Standing balancing activities, such as standing on one leg, can help you improve your balance and core strength by helping you stand on your own two feet. These can be made more difficult by employing a resistance band or holding onto a stationary surface while performing the exercise.

6.Twists, while seated, are an excellent workout for improving flexibility and building strength in the abdominal muscles (obliques). Place your feet level on the ground in front of you and rotate your torso to one side while sitting on a chair. Hold this position for a few seconds before switching sides.

Increase your core strength and general health as a senior by including some of the best core exercises in your regular workout routine. Remember that you should begin your workouts leisurely and progressively raise the intensity and difficulty of your routines as your strength increases.

Adjustments and Variations Made for Individuals with Varying Physical Capabilities

Adjustments and Progressions for People of Varying Degrees of Physical Fitness:

1.Beginners can alter planks by executing them on their forearms or knees on the ground. Planks are an excellent exercise for building core strength. To advance, consider attempting side planks or lifting one leg or arm at a time while holding the plank position.

2.Bridges: Bridges can be adapted so beginners can perform them with both feet planted on the ground or with an object such as a ball or cushion placed between the knees to increase the difficulty level. To advance, you can do bridges with one leg at a time or wrap a resistance band over your thighs.

3.To execute a modified version of the bird dog suitable for beginners, perform the exercise on your hands and knees while extending one leg. You can make the movement more challenging by wrapping a resistance band around your ankles or executing it while standing on a stability ball.

4.Wall Sits an exercise that can be modified for beginners by shortening the time spent in the position. Practice while holding weights or standing on one leg to advance your training.

5.Standing Balance: Standing balancing exercises can be modified for beginners by having them grab onto a sturdy surface or stand with their feet hip-width apart. Exercise on an unsteady surface or with a resistance band to advance your fitness level.

6.For those just starting, it's best to alter seated twists by limiting their range of motion. Try performing the exercise while holding a weight or lifting your feet off the ground to advance your training.

Always pay attention to what your body tells you and adapt your workouts accordingly. If you are experiencing pain or discomfort while exercising, you should immediately stop and speak with a medical expert.

Chapter 5

Bringing It All Together: Developing Your Core Workout Strategies and Techniques

Exercise is the topic of, which can be found here.

This chapter will review the various components of a comprehensive core workout for older adults. Create a complex and effective core-focused workout regimen by combining the most effective core exercises and adapting those exercises to your current level of fitness. This will allow you to target your entire core more effectively.

While designing your core workout, the following stages are some guidelines to follow:

1.Start with a light warm-up consisting of dynamic stretching and low-intensity aerobic exercises like marching in place or riding a stationary bike. This will get your muscles ready for the workout ahead.

2.Pick your workouts: Choose a variety of core exercises that target the abs, lower back, and obliques. Each of these areas should be worked on separately. You can pick and choose from the best core exercises described in **Chapter 4** and adapt them to suit your current fitness level.

3.Set your sets and reps: Select the number of sets and repetitions you will perform for each exercise. The recommended starting range for beginners is 1-2 sets with 10-12 repetitions, and they should gradually extend this range as their strength improves.

4.The recommended amount of rest time between sets is thirty to sixty seconds, depending on the intensity of the workout.

5.The final portion of your workout should consist of a cool-down with static stretching and activities focusing on deep breathing.

You can design a core workout unique to your fitness level and objectives if you follow these steps and pay attention to what your body says. Keep in mind that you should improve gradually and that you should challenge yourself as your strength increases.

How to Create a Workout That Is Balanced Around Your Core

It is essential to target all sections of your core when developing a balanced core workout. These areas include your abdominal muscles, lower back, and oblique muscles. The following are some suggestions that will assist you in developing a balanced core workout:

1.Pick a wide range of exercises: Choose a variety of core workouts that focus on different areas of your abdominal region. Planks are great for targeting your abdominal muscles, bridges are great for targeting your lower back, and side planks are great for targeting your obliques.

2.Exercises that challenge your core stability, like planks, and exercises that increase your core mobility, such as twists, should be incorporated into your workout routine. Pay attention to both strength and mobility.

3.Add progressions: As you gain strength, raise the difficulty of your workouts by performing more repetitions, sets, or resistance. Incorporate progressions.

4.Your core workout should be balanced with other exercises that target different body parts, such as strength training activities for your upper body and lower body, as well as cardiovascular workouts. Remember to include these other types of exercises in your workout routine.

5.You must pay attention to your body and make any necessary adjustments or progressions to your workout routine based on what it tells you. If you are experiencing pain or discomfort while exercising, you should immediately stop and speak with a medical expert.

You can construct a balanced core workout that targets all parts of your core and helps you attain your fitness goals if you follow these recommendations and customize your routine to your current fitness level.

Examples of Exercise Routines Suitable for Many Degrees of Fitness

You can construct your core workout from scratch, but here are some sample programs that are appropriate for different fitness levels that you can use as a starting point

Beginning Workout:

1. Two intervals of thirty seconds each of marching in place

2. Two circuits of 10-15 seconds in the plank position.

3. Bridge: Two sets of ten to twelve reps

4. Two sets of 10-12 repetitions for the dead bug exercise

5. Two sets of ten to twelve reps on each side of the standing side bend.

Exercises for the Intermediate Level:

1. Two intervals of thirty seconds each of marching in place

2.Three sets of 20-30 seconds in the plank position

3.Two sets of twenty to thirty seconds on each side for the side plank

4.Three sets of 10-12 reps should be performed for the reverse crunch.

5.Two sets of 10–12 reps on each side for the Russian twist.

Workout for the Advanced:

1.Two sets of thirty seconds each for high knees.

2.Three sets of 10-12 reps on each side for the plank with leg lift exercise

3.Two sets of 10 to 12 repetitions on either side of the side plank with a leg lift

4.Three sets of ten to twelve repetitions on each side for the bicycle crunch

5.2 sets of 10–12 repetitions for the medicine ball slam.

Always pay attention to your body and make sure you alter exercises appropriately based on your current level of fitness. This will help you avoid injury. To achieve the highest possible level of health and fitness advantages from your entire fitness regimen, it is essential to include a variety of different types of activities, including cardio and strength training.

Chapter 6

Maintaining Your Core Strength is Covered

When you've worked hard to develop a strong core, the next step is to keep it that way so you can keep reaping the advantages of your hard work. Here are some pointers to keep in mind if you want to keep your core strength:

1.Maintain your consistency: Maintaining your consistency is essential if you want to keep your core strength. Your goal should be to conduct core workouts at least twice or three times a week.

2.Step up the intensity: As your strength improves, you should step up the intensity of your workouts by performing additional repetitions, sets, or increasing the resistance.

3.To keep your workouts interesting and challenging for you, try combining new exercises or different types of activities you are already familiar with.

4.Note that your core workouts should be balanced with exercises that target other sections of your body, such as strength training and cardiovascular activity. Ignoring your other muscles is not a good idea.

5.Listen to your body: If you experience any pain or discomfort while exercising, make adjustments to your routine or stop altogether as appropriate. If the discomfort lasts for an extended period, you should seek medical attention.

You can keep your core strength for as long as you like if you follow these suggestions and make core workouts a consistent part of your workout regimen. This will allow you to continue reaping the benefits of having a strong core.

Suggestions to Help You Maintain Your Workout Routine

Keeping up with a fitness routine might be difficult, but the following are some suggestions that can assist you in remaining consistent:

1.Make sure that your goals can be accomplished and are in line with both your capabilities and your timetable before you set them. Your workouts should begin slowly and gradually build in both intensity and duration as you progress.

2.Develop a routine by outlining your workouts in advance and noting the times and locations on your calendar or in your planner. Consider your time spent exercising to be just as important as any other appointment or commitment you have.

3.Locate a workout partner: Exercising with a friend or member of the family will help keep you accountable while also making your exercises more enjoyable.

4.Change things up: If you want to keep your workouts interesting, try switching things up by doing different types of exercises or routines, such as taking dance classes or participating in outdoor activities.

5.Acknowledge and appreciate your development and accomplishments, no matter how minor they may seem, and do so often. Enjoy your victories. This can serve as a source of motivation for you to keep up with your fitness routine.

6.Be gentle to yourself; don't berate yourself if you skip a workout or have a bad day. Instead, treat yourself with compassion. Keep in mind that maintaining consistency is essential, so simply get back on track the next day.

You can improve your odds of sticking to your exercise regimen and attaining your fitness objectives by implementing these recommendations into your regular practice.

Preventing Injuries and Handling Pain

When beginning or continuing an exercise routine, some people experience injuries and pain regularly; nevertheless, there are numerous techniques to prevent injuries and manage discomfort.

1.Always make sure to warm up before you exercise to improve the amount of blood flowing to your muscles and get them ready for the activities ahead.

2.Always be sure to use the correct form when exercising, as this will help you avoid injury and get the most out of your workouts. Get the advice of a trained fitness professional if you are unsure how to perform an activity correctly.

3.Increase the level of your workouts gradually and avoid going straight into strenuous workouts. To avoid damage and give your body time to adjust to the new demands that exercise places on it, you should gradually increase the intensity and duration of your workouts.

4.Listen to your body: If you experience any pain or discomfort while exercising, make adjustments to your routine or stop altogether as appropriate. If you have sustained an injury, you will need to give your body time to heal while you rest.

5. Integrate rest days into your schedule because rest is necessary for healing and preventing injuries. Use rest days as part of your exercise routine to allow your body to recuperate and reduce the risk of overuse problems.

6.Managing discomfort: If you suffer pain while exercising or afterward, you should think about utilizing cold or heat therapy, stretching, or massage to help you manage the pain and speed up your recovery. Pain relievers available without a prescription may also be beneficial; however, before taking any drug, it is important to discuss your treatment options with a qualified medical expert.

You can avoid injury and better manage discomfort if you follow these guidelines, which will allow you to continue reaping the benefits of a consistent exercise routine.

How to Keep Tabs on Your Advancement

It is crucial to keep track of your progress to assist you in maintaining your motivation and achieving your fitness goals. The following are some methods you can monitor your progress:

1.Maintain a notebook: Maintain a journal to keep track of your workouts, including the exercises you complete, the number of sets and reps, as well as how you feel both during and after the workout. This can make it easier for you to recognize how far you've come over time and point out places where you could improve.

2.Take measurements: It is important to take measurements of your body at regular intervals, including your waist circumference, body weight, and the amount of body fat that you have. Even if the number on the scale doesn't budge, you may still show progress and measure changes in your body composition with this method.

3.Use technology: Install fitness tracking applications on your smartphone or wearable devices, such as an Apple Watch or a Fitbit, to keep tabs on your activity level, heart rate, and the number of calories you burn. A good number of these devices also provide you the ability to monitor your development over time.

4.In addition to monitoring your physical development, it is important to establish performance goals. Some examples of performance goals include increasing the number of repetitions or sets that you are capable of performing or decreasing the amount of time it takes you to finish a workout.

5.Honor your achievements and the significant steps you've taken along the path by holding celebrations. This can make it easier for you to maintain your motivation and emphasize the positive adjustments you're making in your life.

You can keep yourself motivated and see how far you've come towards achieving your fitness objectives if you track your progress using these several methods.

Conclusion

I want to congratulate you on taking the initial step toward constructing a robust and healthy core. It is never too late for a senior to begin an exercise routine and improve their general health and well-being; in fact, doing so is never too late. The ability to maintain balance, stability, and mobility requires core strength, which can also assist you to accomplish activities of daily living with greater ease and self-assurance.

We have discussed in this book the significance of core strength for seniors, how to evaluate the level of core strength you now possess, and how to plan and carry out an exercise regimen that is both secure and productive. To further assist you in getting started, we have included a selection of different core exercises as well as example programs.

Keep in mind that developing core strength requires time and effort, but that the benefits more than justify the investment. You can improve the quality of your life as you age while also maintaining your independence if you include core exercises as part of your regular fitness program and adhere to the ideas and guidelines contained in this book.

We are grateful that you have decided to use "Strong at Sixty" as your resource for improving your fitness and core strength. On behalf of both of us, we hope that your new workout routine is a success!

Conclusions and Recommendations Regarding Core Exercises for the Elderly

Seniors need to engage in core workouts if they want to keep their bodies strong, balanced, and healthy. As we become older, the muscles in our core can begin to atrophy, which can result in a variety of health difficulties, including poor posture, back discomfort, and balance problems. You may improve your general health and well-being while also maintaining your independence into your later years if you make core workouts a regular part of your fitness routine.

It is essential to get started cautiously and steadily build up the intensity of your workouts as well as the number of times you perform them. Always pay attention to your body and stop what you're doing if it starts to hurt or make you uncomfortable. It is always best to talk with your doctor before beginning a new exercise regimen, especially if you have any preexisting medical conditions or worries about your health.

It is important to keep in mind that developing a solid foundation is a process, not an end goal. The rewards are worth the effort, even though seeing results takes time and requires consistency. You may improve the quality of your life and maintain your strength and health far into your elderly years if you perform core exercises daily and adhere to the suggestions provided in this book.

Maintaining Our Strength During the Whole Process

Maintaining one's strength over an extended period calls for dedication and perseverance. You must continue to exercise consistently and include a wide range of exercises in your regimen if you want to keep your core strength as you become older. These are some tips for remaining strong:

1.Change things up: If you want to keep your workouts exciting and varied, try out a variety of different forms of activities, such as yoga, Pilates, weight training, and cardiovascular activity.

2.Locate a workout partner; doing exercise with someone else can help keep you motivated and accountable for your progress.

3.Maintain a steady routine: your goal should be to get at st thirty minutes of exercise five days each week. Make it a habit to do it every day, just like brushing your teeth or doing the laundry.

4.Relax and recuperate: Ensure that you give your body enough time to recuperate between sessions of exercise. Get lots of rest and take days off when you feel you need them.

5.Pay attention to your body and stop exercising if you start to feel any pain or discomfort. Instead, go to a medical professional. You should challenge yourself, but not to the point where you risk getting hurt.

It is important to keep in mind that the key to maintaining your strength over the long term is to make adjustments to your lifestyle that promote your general health and well-being. You may maintain your strength and good health far into your senior years if you make core workouts a regular part of your regimen and if you follow the advice in this article.

APPENDIX

FURTHER EXERCISES FOR SENIORS

Crunches while seated

Crunches performed while seated are a useful workout for senior citizens since they help to build core strength and stability. The following is a description of how to perform sitting crunches:

1.Take a seat on a solid chair with your feet planted firmly on the ground and your knees bent slightly.

2.Put your palms down on your thighs and rest your hands there with the backs of your hands facing up.

3.To activate the core muscles in y body, draw your belly button in towards your spine.

4.Lean back gently while ensuring that your back is completely straight and that your shoulders are completely relaxed.

5.Exhale, then bring your hands closer to your knees as you pull your chest towards your knees, continuing to do so as you lift your chest.

6.The crunch should be held for one to two seconds, after which the person should inhale and slowly return to the beginning posture.

7.Continue in this manner for 10–15 repetitions.

Keep in mind that your motions should be slow and under control, and you shouldn't rely on momentum to help you get higher. If you discover that this exercise is too simple for you, you can increase the level of resistance by holding a light weight in each hand.

Tilting of the Pelvis

Pelvic tilts are a low-impact exercise that seniors can do to help increase both their core strength and their flexibility. The following is a description of how to conduct pelvic tilts:

1.Lay on your back with your knees bent and your feet flat on the ground, keeping the distance between them equal to the width of your hips.

2.Put your hands on your side with the palms facing down. Your arms should be by your sides.

3.To activate the core muscles in your body, draw your belly button towards your spine.

4.Exhale, then press your lower back firmly into the ground as you lift your pelvis and gradually tilt it upward.

5.After keeping the tilt for one to two seconds, let out an inhale before releasing the tilt.

6.As you exhale, softly incline your pelvis downward while simultaneously arching your lower back a little bit.

7.After keeping the tilt for one to two seconds, let out an inhale before releasing the tilt.

8.Continue to perform 10–15 repeats of the sequence.

Keep in mind that your motions should be slow and under control, and you should try to avoid arching your back too much. Stop the activity immediately and make an appointment to see a medical professional if you start to feel any discomfort or pain in your back.

Bird Dogs

The exercise known as "bird dogs" is excellent for senior citizens since it helps increase core strength, stability, and balance. The following is the correct way to execute bird dogs:

1.Begin by getting down on your hands and knees, positioning your hands so that they are immediately under your shoulders and your knees so that they are squarely under your hips.

2.To activate the core muscles in your body, draw your belly button towards your spine.

3.Lift your left leg behind you and extend it out in front of you so that both are parallel to the ground. At the same time, extend your right arm out in front of you so that it is parallel to the ground.

4.After holding the position for two to three seconds, you should then slowly lower your arm and leg.

5.Repeat on the opposite side, this time reaching out with your left arm and your right leg.

6.Switch sides after every ten to fifteen repetitions.

Keep in mind that your motions should be slow and under control, and you should steer clear of arching your back or lifting your leg too far. You can alter the exercise such that you perform it on your forearms and knees instead of your wrists and knees if you experience any discomfort or soreness in either of those areas.

Knee Raises

Seniors can benefit from the core strength and hip flexibility that comes from performing knee raises, an activity that is both simple and effective. The following is a description of how to conduct knee raises:

1. You should stand with your feet slightly wider than your hips apart and your arms by your sides.

2. To activate the core muscles in your body, draw your belly button towards your spine.

3. Raise the right knee towards the center of your chest while maintaining a flexed foot position and a straight back position.

4. Maintain the position for two to three seconds, and then slowly bring your leg back down to its starting position.

5. Repeat on the opposite side, this time bringing your left knee closer to your chest as you do so.

6. Switch sides after every ten to fifteen repetitions.

It is important to keep in mind that your motions should be slow and under control, and you should avoid pushing forward or utilizing momentum to lift your leg. If you experience any discomfort or soreness in your hips or knees while executing the exercise, you may wish to adjust it such that you complete it while seated on a stable chair.

Russian Twists Performed While Sitting

Seniors can benefit greatly from seated Russian twists, which are excellent workout that helps increase core strength as well as stability and mobility. The following is a description of how to accomplish seated Russian twists:

1.Take a seat on a solid chair with your feet planted firmly on the ground and your knees bent slightly.

2.Put your palms together on your chest and spread your elbows out to the sides of your body.

3.To activate the core muscles in your body, draw your belly button towards your spine.

4.Exhale as you twist your torso to the right from the waist while maintaining a straight back and rotating your upper body to the right.

5.After holding the twist for one to two seconds, inhale as you circle back to the center of the room.

6.Exhale as you twist your torso to the left starting from your waist while maintaining a straight back position. Rotate your upper body clockwise.

7.After holding the twist for one to two seconds, inhale as you circle back to the center of the room.

8.Continue to perform 10–15 repeats of the sequence. Keep in mind that your movements should be slow and under control, and you should steer clear of using momentum to twist your torso. If you experience any discomfort or pain in your back or neck while performing the exercise, you can alter it by reducing the resistance or decreasing the range of motion you perform.

Planks

Planks are an exercise that can assist seniors to improve their core strength, stability, and posture. They are also demanding workouts that can be beneficial. The following is a guide for how to perform planks:

1. Put your hands on the ground just behind your shoulders and place your feet hip-width apart. Assume a push-up position.

2. To activate the core muscles in your body, draw your belly button towards your spine

. 3. Reduce your weight on your forearms while maintaining a position in which your elbows are directly under your shoulders.

4.Pull your knees up in your chest and increase your legs at the back of you in order that there's a directly line going for walks out of your head in your heels.

5. Maintaining a straight back and level hips while you hold the plank posture for 10 to 30 seconds is a good goal.

6. After releasing the plank and resting for a few seconds, perform two or three sets of exercises. It is important to keep in mind that your motions should be steady and controlled and that you should avoid allowing your hips to sag or lifting them too high. You can adjust the exercise so that you perform it on your knees rather than your toes if you experience any discomfort or soreness in your wrists or shoulders. This will allow you to reduce the strain placed on those areas.

Side Planks

Seniors can benefit from a hard yet effective exercise called side planks, which can assist increase core strength as well as stability and balance. The following is a description of how to accomplish side planks:

1. Place yourself on your side with your legs extended straight out in front of you and your feet piled one on top of the other.

2. Put your weight on your elbow and keep your forearm flat on the ground while positioning your bending arm such that it is directly under your shoulder.

3. To activate the core muscles in your body, draw your belly button towards your spine.

4. Raise your hips off the ground and bring your head into a line with your feet, creating a straight line from head to foot.

5. Maintain the side plank posture for ten to thirty seconds, making sure to keep your hips in line with each other and your shoulders stacked on top of each other.

6. After releasing the side plank and taking a short break, you should repeat the exercise on the other side. Keep in mind that your movements should be slow and under control, and you should steer clear of allowing your hips to sag or lean either forward or backward. You can adapt to the exercise by doing it on your forearm and keeping your elbow precisely under your shoulder if you experience any discomfort or soreness in your wrists or shoulders. This will allow the workout to be performed on your forearm.

Dead Bugs

A senior citizen's core strength and stability, as well as their hip and shoulder mobility, can all be improved by the use of dead bugs as an excellent kind of exercise. The following is the correct way to perform dead bugs:

1. When you lie on your back, bring your arms up towards the sky and bend your legs so that they make a

right angle with your torso. Position your knees so that they are directly over your hips.

2. With a flat back on the floor and a strong core engagement, move your right arm and left leg toward the ground in a slow and controlled manner.

4. After your arm and leg are hovering a few inches above the ground, you should pause the movement and return to the starting position.

5. Repeat the motion on the opposite side, this time bringing your left arm and right leg closer to the floor.

6. Keep going, changing sides for the next ten to fifteen repetitions. It is important to keep in mind that your motions should be slow and under control and that you should avoid arching your back or allowing your legs to descend too low. If you experience any stiffness or pain in your lower back while performing the exercise, you can

adjust it by lowering only one limb at a time instead of both at the same time.

Superman Pose

The Superman stance is an excellent workout for senior citizens since it can assist improve core strength and posture while also activating the back and gluteal muscles. The Superman posture can be achieved by following these steps

1.Position yourself so that you are lying face down on a mat or other cushioned surface with your arms stretched out in front of you and your legs extended straight behind you.

2. To activate the core muscles in your body, draw your belly button towards your spine. 3. Raise your arms, torso, and legs off the ground and assume a "superman" pose by doing so. 4. After holding the position for two to

three seconds, slowly release it and return your body to the starting position.

5. Continue in this manner for 10–15 repetitions. Keep in mind that your motions should be slow and under control, and you should avoid raising too much weight or arching your back an excessive amount. If you experience any stiffness or pain in your lower back, you should adapt the exercise so that you are only lifting one of your arms or legs at a time rather than both at the same time.

Full Planks

Full planks are a demanding exercise that can help improve core strength, posture, and overall stability for seniors. The following is a description of how to complete full planks:

1. Put your hands on the ground just behind your shoulders and place your feet hip-width apart. Assume a push-up position.

2.Pull your knees up on your chest and enlarge your legs in the back of you in order that there may be a immediately line strolling out of your head on your heels.

3,. Maintaining a straight back and level hips while you hold the plank posture for 10 to 30 seconds is a good goal.

4. After releasing the plank and resting for a few seconds, perform two or three sets of exercise. It is important to keep in mind that your motions should be steady and controlled and that you should avoid allowing your hips to sag or lifting them too high.

You can adjust the exercise so that you perform it on your knees rather than your toes if you experience any discomfort or soreness in your wrists or shoulders. This will allow you to reduce the strain placed on those areas. Full planks require more strength and stability than modified planks do, so it's important to work up to this exercise gradually and only perform it if you feel comfortable and confident in your abilities. Modified planks are a great alternative to full planks if you're just getting started with planking.

Crunches on a bicycle

The bicycle crunch is an excellent exercise for seniors that can help improve core strength and coordination, as well as hip and knee mobility. Bicycle crunches are performed on a stationary bicycle. The following is a description of how to conduct bicycle crunches:

1. Position yourself so that you are lying on your back with your hands clasped behind your head and your knees bent at a ninety-degree angle while keeping your feet off the ground.

2. Raise your shoulders off the ground and, at the same time, pull your right elbow in close to your left knee while simultaneously extending your right leg out in a straight line.

4. Bring your left elbow closer to your right knee as you extend your left leg out in a straight line. Then, return to the beginning position and repeat the exercise on the other side.

5. Keep going, changing sides for the next ten to fifteen repetitions. Keep in mind that your movements should be gradual and under control, and you should avoid putting any strain on your neck or allowing your shoulders to round forward. If you feel any discomfort or pain in your neck or back, you may want to alter the exercise by keeping your head and shoulders on the ground while you complete the leg motions solely. This may help alleviate the discomfort or pain.

Climbers of the Mountains

Climbing mountains is a demanding workout that can help seniors improve their core strength, cardiovascular endurance, and hip mobility. The following is the correct form for mountain climbers:

1.To activate the core muscles in your body, draw your belly button towards your spine.

2.Pull your right knee in towards your chest, and then rapidly switch and bring your left knee in towards your chest while extending your right leg back behind you.

3.Keep alternating your legs in a fast hopping action, as though you were running in place while you were in the push-up position.

4.Try to do the exercise for thirty to sixty seconds at a time.

It is important to keep your movements rapid and under control, and you should also avoid allowing your hips to slump or lifting them too high. You can adjust the exercise so that you perform it on your knees rather than your toes if you experience any discomfort or soreness in your wrists or shoulders. This will allow you to reduce the strain placed on those areas. Mountain climbers are a high-impact activity, so it's crucial to pay attention to your body and only practice the exercise if you're sure you can handle it and are comfortable with the challenges it presents.

Side Jackknives

Jackknives to the side are a fantastic workout for seniors because they work the oblique muscles that are located on the sides of the core. Performing side jackknives can be done as follows:

1.Position yourself so that you are lying on your side with your legs stretched out in front of you and your lower arm supporting your head.

2.To activate the core muscles in your body, draw your belly button towards your spine.

3.Raise your upper arm towards your feet as you lift your legs off the ground and bring them in towards your chest at the same time.

4.After pausing at the peak, begin lowering your legs and arms back down to the starting position in a controlled manner.

5.Continue in this manner for 10–15 repetitions on one side, then swap sides and continue in this manner.

It is important to make sure that your motions are slow and under control, and that you do not allow your shoulders to round or your knees to sink too much. If you have any discomfort or pain in your neck or back, you can alter the workout by keeping your head and shoulders on the ground and lifting only your legs. This will allow you to focus on strengthening your legs without aggravating your neck or back.

Because side jackknives need a fair level of stability and balance, it is crucial to work up to this exercise gradually, and you should only practice it if you feel comfortable and secure in your capabilities.

Spiderman Planks

The core, shoulders, and hip flexors are all targeted effectively with spiderman planks, which are a hard exercise for seniors. The following is a description of how to accomplish spiderman planks:

1.To begin, get into the plank position by placing both hands on the ground immediately under your shoulders and keeping your feet hip-width apart.

2.To activate the core muscles in your body, draw your belly button towards your spine.

3.While maintaining your foot off the ground, bring your right knee up to meet your right elbow.

4.Take a little pause, and then bring your right leg back to where it was at the beginning of the exercise.

5.Do the same movement on the opposite side, this time bringing your left knee to your left elbow.

6.Keep going, changing sides for the next ten to fifteen repetitions.

It is important to keep in mind that your motions should be steady and controlled and that you should avoid allowing your hips to sag or lifting them too high. You can adjust the exercise so that you perform it on your knees rather than your toes if you experience any discomfort or soreness in your wrists or shoulders.

This will allow you to reduce the strain placed on those areas. Because spiderman planks involve a fair level of stability and balance, it is vital to work up to this exercise gradually, and you should only execute it if you feel comfortable and secure in your capabilities.

The Advantages that Comes with Having a Solid Core for Seniors

For seniors to keep their general health and well-being in good shape, they must have a robust core. Exercises that focus on the core can assist improve one's balance, stability, and posture, as well as lower one's risk of injury and falling over. A strong core can also help seniors conduct activities of daily living more smoothly and with less pain or discomfort. This is especially helpful for those who have limited mobility. Seniors can enjoy the benefits of a stronger and healthier body by making core exercises a daily part of their routine and reaping the rewards of a stronger and healthier body. It is essential to keep in mind that you should begin with low intensity, employ the correct form, and pay attention to what your body tells you to do to prevent damage or discomfort. Seniors have the potential to enhance their core strength and live a life that is healthier and more active if they are consistent and dedicated.